BEAT STRESS

BULLET GUIDE

Mac Bride

Hodder Education, 338 Euston Road, London NW1 3BH

Hodder Education is an Hachette UK company

First published in UK 2011 by Hodder Education

This edition published 2011

Copyright © 2011 Mac Bride

The moral rights of the author have been asserted

Database right Hodder Education (makers)

Artworks (internal and cover): Peter Lubach
Cover concept design: Two Associates

British Library Cataloguing in Publication Data: a catalogue record for this title is available from the British Library.

10 9 8 7 6 5 4 3 2 1

The publisher has used its best endeavours to ensure that any website addresses referred to in this book are correct and active at the time of going to press. However, the publisher and the author have no responsibility for the websites and can make no guarantee that a site will remain live or that the content will remain relevant, decent or appropriate.

The publisher has made every effort to mark as such all words which it believes to be trademarks. The publisher should also like to make it clear that the presence of a word in the book, whether marked or unmarked, in no way affects its legal status as a trademark.

Every reasonable effort has been made by the publisher to trace the copyright holders of material in this book. Any errors or omissions should be notified in writing to the publisher, who will endeavour to rectify the situation for any reprints and future editions.

Hachette UK's policy is to use papers that are natural, renewable and recyclable products and made from wood grown in sustainable forests. The logging and manufacturing processes are expected to conform to the environmental regulations of the country of origin.

www.hoddereducation.co.uk

Typeset by Stephen Rowling/Springworks

Printed in Spain

Contents

About the author

Mac Bride saw his first book published in 1982, and since then he has written more than 120 books on various aspects of programming, computer applications, the internet, language books for house buyers, green issues and other topics. As well as writing, he has edited and typeset books on subjects ranging from marketing through *feng shui* to Postmodernism.

In his roles as teacher, freelancer, father and chair of governors, he has learned a lot about stress and claims to have now got it pretty well beaten. When not at his desk, he can be found in the kitchen, or the cinema, or playing with his grandchildren.

Introduction

We all come under pressure, to a greater or lesser extent, at times. Some pressures are good: targets, deadlines and the desire to shine can motivate us to perform better. But if the pressure is too great it becomes a problem and we suffer from stress.

Is there anything we can do to help ourselves? Yes. We can improve our ability to cope with pressure by:

* learning simple relaxation techniques
* getting into better sleep habits
* taking a little more care of what we eat and drink
* managing our time and energies better
* setting realistic targets for ourselves
* recognizing what really matters.

This book will help with all of these things.

1 What is stress?

Pressure and stress

We all come under pressure at times, and most of the time we cope quite happily with it. Some of us thrive on it. But if the pressure is too great, or goes on for too long, it becomes a problem and we suffer from stress.

This chapter looks at common **sources of stress**, the positive and negative effects of performing under pressure, how stress affects body chemistry and the main ways of dealing with stress.

Stress is not the pressure itself, but your **reaction** to it – which means that you can control your stress.

Stress is not the pressure itself, but your reaction to it

* The pressures that cause stress are known as **stressors**.
* Stressors can be internal – from within us – or external – from any aspect of our lives.
* Up to a point, stress can be a good thing.
* Stress affects our body chemistry.
* We may need **professional help** to cope with stress.

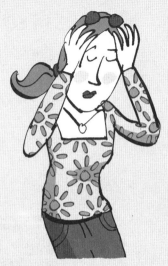

● '...and then he said I could control my own stress, so that's another thing to worry about!'

Sources of stress

Our stressors can be **internal** or **external**.

Internal stressors

* Unrealistic expectations of self
* Attitudes to problems
* Poor time management
* Over-worrying
* Low self-esteem

External stressors

* Too much work
* Not enough money
* Poor housing
* Illness – yours or that of a loved one
* Difficult relationships

4

Pleasant as well as unpleasant changes in life can be sources of stress.

Duration

How long pressure lasts is important. We can take quite a lot of pressure if we know that there will be an end to it – the project will be finished one day, the loved one will recover from the illness, the kids will go back to school soon.

Lighter pressures can cause stress if there's no end in sight. Things do not have to be dramatically bad to be stressful – it's enough that they are not good and there is little prospect of change.

> **'I try to take one day at a time, but sometimes several days attack me at once.'**
>
> Jennifer Yane

Performing under pressure

Some pressure is good. If no one – neither you nor anyone else – cares whether, when or how something is done, it probably won't get done.

Targets, deadlines and other pressures can motivate you to perform better up to a point, but beyond that, pressures can reduce performance.

The levels of performance under pressure

1 **Why bother?** No pressure, no motivation, little gets done.
2 **Getting into gear.** Motivated to do things, ticking over gently.
3 **Performing well.** Coping with the pressures and feeling good about it.
4 **Feeling the strain.** Everything gets done, but it's exhausting.
5 **Overstressed.** In a downward spiral, where stress reduces performance.
6 **It's too much!**

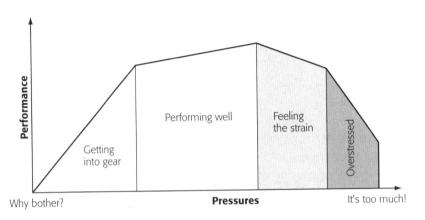

Performance

Why bother?

Getting
into gear

Performing well

Feeling
the strain

Overstressed

Pressures

It's too much!

● The levels of performance under pressure

Pressures **change over time**. In many organizations, the pressure is higher at certain times of the year. People who are 'performing well' most of the year will be 'feeling the strain' or 'overstressed' at peak times.

Stress and body chemistry

Stress affects our body chemistry. It's all part of the 'fight or flight' response to danger – inherited from our ancient ancestors.

* Adrenalin and other stress hormones prepare our bodies for vigorous action.
* The heart beats faster, breathing speeds up, glucose and fat are released into the blood to power the muscles, and blood pressure rises.
* The blood clots more easily, digestion slows down, the pupils dilate, and we start to sweat.

'He who smiles rather than rages is always the stronger.'

Japanese proverb

Stress makes us ready to fight or run, but if we don't do either, our body chemistry is out of whack. The unused fat may clog our arteries, which makes a stroke or heart attack more likely. Stomach ulcers and other digestive problems are also common outcomes.

Chronic work stress can increase our risk of disease, but lifestyle is a key factor, so we can help ourselves.

● The body prepares for fight or flight

What can I do about it?

The short answer is 'quite a lot'.

You can improve your ability to cope with pressure by:

* learning simple **relaxation techniques**
* getting into better **sleep habits**
* taking a little more care of what you **eat** and **drink**.

You can reduce the pressures you create for yourself by:

* **managing** your time and energies better
* setting **realistic** targets for yourself
* recognizing what **really** matters.

I can't cope any more. It's all too much.

When to seek professional help

Self-help will sometimes not be enough. Severe stress may need medical intervention and/or professional **counselling**.

If stress is significantly affecting your health or your ability to cope with your job or your everyday life, **see your GP** or family physician. Recognizing that you have a stress problem, and getting other people to recognize it, is an essential first step in getting to grips with it.

Recognizing that you have a stress problem is an essential first step in getting to grips with it

2 The signs of stress

How do I know if I'm stressed?

People are different and react to pressures in different ways. When some people are stressed, the signs are obvious to themselves and to others around them. But not everyone shows **telltale signs**, especially in the early stages, and stress – like so many problems – can be dealt with most easily if caught early.

> **'Reality is the leading cause of stress amongst those in touch with it.'**
> Lily Tomlin

People react to pressures in different ways

Stress can affect what people do, what they say, and what they think and feel. It may affect, among other things:

* performance at work
* relations with friends and family
* appetite, eating and drinking habits
* sleep patterns
* health.

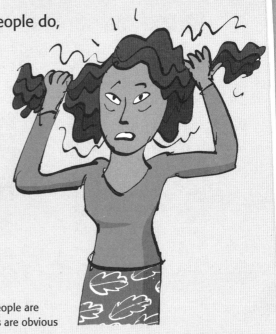

● When some people are stressed, the signs are obvious

Stress and personality type

Psychologists tell us that there are **two types of personality** when it comes to coping with stress, and we may be completely one or the other, or a mixture of the two. Here are ten key traits of these two personality types.

Tick those that you feel apply to you, then count up how many you have in each set. The more Type A you are, the more likely you are to suffer from stress. Type B personalities cope better.

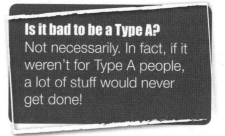

Is it bad to be a Type A?
Not necessarily. In fact, if it weren't for Type A people, a lot of stuff would never get done!

Type A

- ☐ Competitive
- ☐ Impatient
- ☐ Works hard, and fast
- ☐ Perfectionist
- ☐ Always on time, or early
- ☐ Will work late and/or take work home
- ☐ Will try to do several things at once
- ☐ Speaks quickly and interrupts slow speakers
- ☐ Does not express feelings
- ☐ Few hobbies/social activities

Type B

- ☐ Laid back
- ☐ Patient
- ☐ Slow, steady worker
- ☐ Near enough is good enough
- ☐ Often late
- ☐ Works the hours, and no more
- ☐ Won't try to multi-task
- ☐ Listens to others
- ☐ Open about own feelings
- ☐ Active social life

Self-imposed stress...

Your personality doesn't just affect how you react to stress; it may also create stresses.

The classic Type A personality needs to be **in control** of their life and environment at all times, and reacts to any perceived attempt to challenge this control. For example, traffic jams or delayed trains that threaten to make them late for meetings can generate feelings of anger, out of proportion to how much being late really matters. It's the **anger** that stresses them, not the delay.

'Don't sweat the small stuff – and it's all small stuff.'

Kristine and Richard Carlson

... and how to reduce it

Type A behaviour is **largely learned**, and can be unlearned. Next time you feel yourself getting uptight, angry or frustrated about a delay or problem, ask yourself:

✳ Is the level of my response appropriate? It may be. But if it isn't, then you need to pull yourself back.
✳ Does my response help? If not, is there anything else I could do that would either help solve the problem or enable me to cope with it better?
✳ Could I have avoided this situation? Are there lessons to be learned for the future?

Type A behaviour is largely learned, and can be unlearned

Recognizing the symptoms: behaviour

We all of us are aware of being stressed at times, and we cope with it as part of life's normal flow. We may not realize when stress has become **a problem** for us, and be even less aware when others are suffering.

What's changed?

We are all different, and everything is relative. When thinking about your own or other people's **symptoms**, pay attention to what has changed. Compared to six months or a year ago, has there been a change in the person's work, relationships or other key aspect of their life? Have symptoms developed since then?

Possible signs of stress

High stress levels can show up in attitudes and behaviour.

Some signs may be more visible to the **sufferer**:

* poor concentration
* anxiety
* depression
* feeling of lack of control
* feeling unable to cope
* difficulty sleeping.

Some are more likely to be noticed by **other people**:

* hair-trigger temper
* smoking too much
* drinking too much alcohol and/or caffeine
* nervous tics, such as tapping, scratching, or twiddling hair.

Recognizing the symptoms: physical

The impact of the fight-or-flight stress reaction on the body's chemistry can show up in a number of **physical symptoms**. These include:

* headaches or hot flushes
* dry mouth and shaky hands
* chest pain or palpitations
* digestive problems
* loss of sex drive
* eczema or other skin conditions.

Play safe: see your doctor

These symptoms can be caused by stress, but can also arise from other causes. Either way, if you suffer significantly from any of them, **see your doctor**.

22

Stress and health

The high levels of stress hormones **cortisol, noradrenalin** and **adrenalin** can be bad for you.

* **Cortisol** weakens the immune system and reduces the body's ability to fight infections, across a range of diseases from the common cold to arthritis and cancer.
* **Noradrenalin** affects the heart. It constricts blood vessels, which raises blood pressure and makes the heart work harder. If the coronary arteries – the ones that supply blood to the heart – are clogged with plaque, the stress can trigger angina (chest pains) or a full-blown heart attack. Noradrenalin can also cause these arteries to spasm, and may also rupture the plaque causing blockages.
* **Noradrenalin** and **adrenalin** are also known to damage the heart muscles directly, and can cause abnormal heartbeat rhythms, which can be fatal.

3 Diet and exercise

Healthy body, healthy mind

There's a lot of truth in the old saying. Your physical health is important, for your brain is part of your body. It can't do its job properly if it's got the **wrong hormones** and other chemicals washing through it.

Sorting out your health should be one of the first things you do to tackle stress, as it is – normally – within your control, and it can have a quick impact.

It's harder for your mind to function well if your body is in poor condition

Better health

For better bodily health you need to take control in these areas:

* what you eat, and when
* what you drink, and how much
* how much exercise you take
* your sleeping habits.

We'll look at diet and exercise in this section, and cover sleep in the next.

'While we may not be able to control all that happens to us, we can control what happens inside us.'

Benjamin Franklin

Eating well

Try to eat regularly and avoid snacking between meals. Aim for a **balanced diet** – one that will supply your body with the materials it needs – in appropriate quantities. Skipping meals is not a good idea. Without fuel, your body will lack energy and so will your brain.

Your **daily diet** should include:

* fruit and vegetables, for vitamins, minerals and fibre – and fresh is best
* starchy foods such as bread and other cereals, pasta and potatoes, for energy
* meat, fish or alternative sources of proteins, such as beans
* milk for calcium and vitamins.

Help lower stress levels by eating a balanced diet

What not to eat

Stress tends to raise **blood pressure** and **cholesterol levels**, and can affect the digestive system, leading to ulcers or irritable bowel syndrome. Avoid foods that will make any of these worse:

* junk food – typically high in salt, fat and sugar
* high-cholesterol foods such as egg yolk, butter, cheese and fatty meat
* anything with a high level of refined sugar – it can mess with your blood sugar levels and hence your moods.

There is evidence that dark chocolate may help reduce blood pressure, cholesterol and stress hormones. Good news! (But eat small quantities only, or the sugar and fat intake outweighs the benefits.)

Drinking healthily

It's a myth that you need to drink several litres of water a day. You don't. You get most of the water you need from your food and normal drinks. Drink when you are thirsty – but watch your consumption of caffeine and alcohol.

Caffeine is a stimulant that causes the release of adrenalin – the stress hormone – into your system. Limit yourself to **no more than five** coffees, teas or caffeine-rich soft drinks a day. It's also addictive, so if you are over that level, reduce gradually to avoid withdrawal symptoms.

Top tip
If you have to work overlong hours to meet a deadline, don't rely on caffeine to keep you going. Take a short nap or relaxation break when you start to droop. You'll work better, and faster, afterwards.

Alcohol, in moderate quantities, can be good for you and can be part of relaxing with friends, but keep **within the limits** (2–3 units a day for women, 3–4 units for men):

❋ It is a mood enhancer, so if you are already down it'll make it worse.
❋ It stimulates the production of adrenalin, adding to feelings of stress.
❋ It interferes with liver function, slowing down the removal of toxins from the blood.
❋ You don't sleep so well after drinking, and don't work so well with a hangover, which may add to stress.

> **'The only way to keep your health is to eat what you don't want, drink what you don't like and do what you'd rather not.'**
> Mark Twain

Exercise is good for you

Why exercise?

* It's good for your heart and blood pressure.
* A physically fit body can cope better with mental stress.
* It improves blood flow to the brain, enabling better thinking.
* It relaxes tense muscles, which helps you sleep.

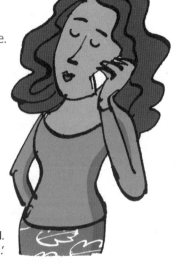

● 'I tried yoga, but got bored. It's more fun being stressed.'

Exercise and brain chemistry

The adrenalin produced by stress prepares your body for **action**, and action will help to bring your chemistry back to normal. Aerobics and other high-energy exercise will burn off excess sugar and fats in the blood, and clear the adrenalin from your system, relieving feelings of **tension** and **frustration**.

During prolonged exercise the body produces **endorphins**, which work directly on the brain. They suppress pain and lift the mood, like morphine but without being addictive. Why are you tired but happy at the end of a run, or a brisk walk, or a hard-fought game? It's partly the sense of achievement, and partly the endorphin high.

Top tip
If all you've done all day is sit at a computer, your brain may be tired but your body will be more than ready for exercise.

How much exercise do I need?

The answer depends upon what you are trying to achieve. For general good health, **30 minutes** of moderate exercise three days a week is the recommended minimum.

Moderate exercise can be walking, cycling, sport, even gardening or housework. What matters is that it raises your heart rate to at least 50 per cent of your maximum, and that you enjoy it so that you keep doing it.

If you are **out of condition**, work up towards it. Start with fairly gentle exercise, for ten minutes (three times) in the first week, then five minutes longer each week to reach 30. And push yourself a bit harder every time.

> ## 'The sovereign invigorator of the body is exercise, and of all the exercises walking is the best.'
> Thomas Jefferson

34

Heart rate targets

You can calculate your maximum heart rate for exercising by subtracting your age from 220. If you are 30 years old, your maximum heart rate would be: 220 − 30 = 190. When exercising, aim for **between 50 and 90 per cent** of the maximum, depending upon what you are trying to achieve.

Maximum heart rate	Fitness level
90% – upper limit	Extreme physical fitness
80%	Respiratory benefits
70%	Endorphins release
60%	Cardiovascular benefits
50% – minimum	General good health

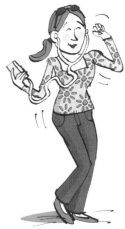

● 'Other people can run a marathon – this is my kind of exercise.'

4 Sleep

Poor sleep and stress

Sleeping badly and stress can be a **vicious circle**. You can't sleep because of stress, and after a bad night you can't perform at your best, so things are more likely to go wrong, which adds to the stress. Then you start to worry because you're not sleeping properly…

But the circle can be broken, and turned around. After a **good night's sleep** you will perform better, your stress levels will go down and you'll sleep better.

The stress > sleeping badly > stress circle can be broken

Breaking the cycle

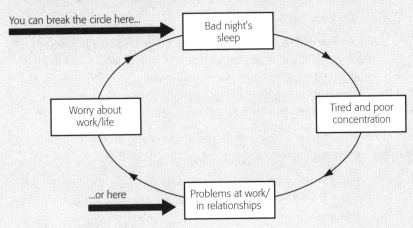

You can break the circle here...

Bad night's sleep

Tired and poor concentration

...or here

Problems at work/ in relationships

Worry about work/life

● Where to break the bad sleep cycle

How much sleep do I need?

There are two main types of sleep:

1 **Rapid Eye Movement (REM) sleep** occurs at intervals throughout the night, and makes up about one-fifth of our sleep. The brain is active, dreaming, and the eyes move rapidly.
2 In **non-REM sleep** the brain is quiet, but the body may move. Non-REM sleep can be light or very deep.

In normal sleep you come to the point of waking several times a night, and may wake fully if disturbed.

Most adults need around **eight hours' sleep** a night, though some need less. As we get older we tend to need less sleep, and wake more often and for longer.

Most adults need around eight hours' sleep a night

Is lack of sleep a real problem?

It depends on how much sleep you are missing. The odd bad night will leave you feeling tired, but otherwise OK.

* If you generally sleep badly, you might:
  » fall asleep during the day
  » find it hard to concentrate
  » find it hard to make decisions
  » be depressed.
* Full-blown insomnia, where you are either not sleeping at all or only for very brief periods, may produce:
  » paranoia
  » hallucinations.

'The amount of sleep required by the average person is five minutes more.'

Wilson Mizener

Your body and sleep

There are a number of **physical reasons** why you may find it hard to fall asleep or sleep well:

* uncomfortable bed
* bedroom too hot/cold/noisy
* lack of exercise during the day
* heavy meal a few hours before bedtime
* hunger
* caffeine up to six hours before bedtime
* alcohol, especially in excess
* stimulants such as slimming tablets or
  illicit drugs such as ecstasy and cocaine.

42

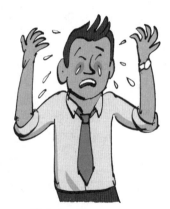

● 'I should never have had that cup of coffee!'

Most of these problems are easily remedied:

* You can greatly improve a **bed** that's too hard with a foam topper; if it's too soft you should replace the mattress.
* If you've had a desk-bound day, take an early-evening walk, or go to a sports club, do yoga, have sex – anything to **move** your muscles and tire your body.
* Take your evening **meal** earlier, or, if it has to be late, then keep it light.
* If you want a hot drink, choose decaff or have hot chocolate or milk, or herbal tea.
* **Cut out** as many **stimulants** as possible from your diet.

> Research has shown that using stress-reducing techniques like these is more effective than sleeping pills at breaking the cycle of insomnia.

Your mind and sleep

Preparing your mind for sleep is as important as preparing your body. Being free from stress and worry is, of course, a major part of that, but **attitudes** and **habits** also make a difference, and you can tackle these separately.

A key part of this is building a **clear association** in your mind between bed and sleep. Don't use your bed as a place to work, surf, watch TV or do anything else you must stay awake for (make an exception for sex).

Don't lie awake worrying: if you are in bed and find you cannot sleep, get up again and do something relaxing. Go back when you feel sleepy.

> **Top tip**
> Siestas, 'power naps' and afternoon snoozes can all be good stress beaters, but avoid them if sleeping at night is a problem.

Bedtime routines

Set yourself a **regular bedtime** – not just the time, but also the **routines** before it.

✳ If you have something on your mind at bedtime, **write it down** and tell yourself you will deal with it in the morning.
✳ **Relax properly** before going to bed. Wind down with an undemanding book or radio or TV programme, or try the relaxation exercises in the next chapter.
✳ **Don't worry** that you must be asleep by a certain time.

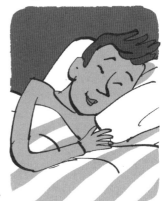

● 'Deal with it in the morning...'

I still can't sleep!

Will medication help?

Sleeping tablets are prescribed far less now than they used to be because they don't really help. They quickly lose their effect as your body gets used to them, so you have to take higher doses; they are addictive; and they can leave you drowsy and grouchy the next day. If you do use them, it should only be as a **short-term measure** to help build better sleep patterns.

Most non-prescription sleeping medicines are based on antihistamine, which will leave you drowsy for some time the next morning, and which loses its effect with prolonged use.

> **Top tip**
> Make sure your bedroom clocks are out of view, so that you don't see the minutes ticking by when you can't sleep.

How about 'natural' remedies?

The **herbal sleep remedies** normally use valerian, which seems to have little effect until you have been taking it regularly for several weeks. (And that may be more to do with establishing sleep routines.)

Rather than resorting to medication, it's probably better to try to get to **the root** of your sleeping problem and find out what works best for you.

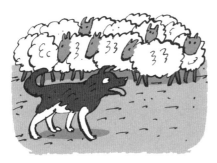

● Counting sheep probably isn't the best remedy for sleeplessness…

'People who say they sleep like a baby usually don't have one.'
Leo J. Burke

5 Relaxation

Make time to relax

Don't say you haven't got time to relax. Relaxing may well **save** you time. Even a **short break** can recharge the batteries and give you the energy to do a lot more work, and do it with a clearer head.

The longer you can spend relaxing the better, but just a few moments is enough, as long as you can relax your body **completely**. In this section you will learn some simple techniques to do just that.

Relaxing may save you time in the long run

> **'For fast-acting relief, try slowing down.'**
> Lily Tomlin

To relax, you need to:

* take time out – ideally at least 15 minutes, though one quick minute can be enough.
* find or create a calm environment
* breathe properly
* lose the tension from your muscles
* defocus your mind.

Taking exercise, enjoying a hobby, eating with friends or watching a movie are also forms of relaxation, but this section looks at techniques for 'the sitting or lying quietly and at peace' type.

Setting the environment

You need **time** and **space** in which to relax, but the time needn't be that long, and you can create the space yourself.

Time

* For deep relaxation, allow at least **15 minutes**.
* Make deep relaxation part of your **daily routine**.
* For **quick relief**, you only need one minute or less.
* Use the quick relief as needed.

You need to be able to switch off completely in this time, and be free from interruptions. This means that you can't take the quick relief while you are driving, but you could do in a traffic jam.

For deep relaxation, allow at least 15 minutes

Space

For deep relaxation, choose:

* somewhere warm and comfortable: ideally flat out, or in a chair where you can recline
* soft lighting or at least some means of shading your eyes
* calm music: partly for itself, partly to help block out other sounds.

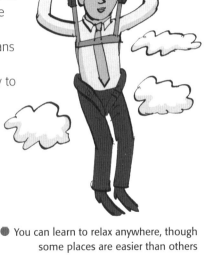

● You can learn to relax anywhere, though some places are easier than others

Breathe easy

During exercise, when the body needs plenty of **oxygen**, you pull air into your lungs by expanding your upper chest. At other times, you normally draw air into your lungs by moving your diaphragm down, which pushes the abdomen out. Under stress, you may breathe by rapid upper chest movement, and this is not good.

Deep, rapid breathing is **hyperventilation**, which flushes too much carbon dioxide out of the blood, making it alkaline. On the other hand, shallow rapid breathing doesn't flush out enough carbon dioxide, and the blood becomes acidic. Neither is good for you!

Breathing properly is a first essential step in getting your body back into balance

54

1-2-3-4, breathe!

Do this as part of a relaxation, or as a **quick tension buster**:

1 Lie down, or sit down and lean back.
2 Rest one hand on your upper chest, and one on your abdomen. As you breathe, notice the movement of your hands.
3 Breathe in slowly, counting to four in your head. Push your abdomen out, so that your diaphragm expands your lungs.
4 Hold in the breath, counting to four.
5 Breathe out slowly, letting your abdomen relax, counting to four.
6 Repeat until you feel calmer. Sometimes it only takes a few cycles to break the build-up of stress.

Top tip
As you breathe, concentrate on making the hand on your abdomen rise up. If only the hand on your chest moves, your breathing is too shallow.

Relax your muscles

It's hard to relax a muscle if you don't know it's tense. With the **progressive muscular relaxation (PMR) technique** you tense muscles first before relaxing them, so that you are aware of the difference. With practice, you can learn to relax muscles quickly, without tensing.

In a full PMR session, all the muscles in your body are tensed and relaxed in turn. Don't be surprised if you fall asleep at the end. If you have things to do, set an alarm before you start – **15 minutes** will be enough to leave you relaxed and refreshed.

Caution!
If you suffer from high blood pressure, or back pain or other muscular problems, check with your GP before trying this.

Simplified PMR

1 Sit comfortably, or lie flat somewhere warm and quiet.
2 Close your eyes.
3 Take each muscle group in turn in this order:
   a right leg
   b left leg
   c right hand and arm
   d left hand and arm
   e abdomen
   f neck and shoulders
   g face.
4 Focus on the muscles, breathe in and squeeze them as hard as you can for eight seconds.
5 Breathe out and relax the muscles.
6 Breathe 1-2-3-4 again, and then repeat for that group.
7 When you have worked through the whole body, stay relaxed for five minutes and picture yourself in a favourite peaceful place.
8 Open your eyes, breathe 1-2-3-4 again, stretch gently and get up slowly.

Letting go quickly

If you practise PMR regularly, you'll become able to relax your muscles **at will**, without tensing. In the meantime, here are two methods of quickly reducing stress levels and calming yourself down.

Method 1: whole body tense and relax

You need 20–30 seconds' time out for this. You can be sitting or standing, but you might want to find a private spot.

1 Clench your fists, toes, buttocks, jaw and all places in between.
2 Breathe in, counting to 4, increasing the tension all the time.
3 Hold the tension for the count of 4.
4 Breathe out, relaxing the muscles slowly, to the count of 4.
5 Repeat if necessary, or if there is time.

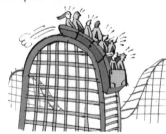

● 'Get off that roller coaster...'

Method 2: instant peace

This is even quicker and less obtrusive, and you could do it in a meeting if tempers and tensions are beginning to climb. This will leave you **calmer** and **clearer**.

1 Close your eyes.
2 Focus on the thing or person that is causing the stress.
3 Say to yourself: 'Stay calm. You can handle this.'
4 Breathe in 1-2-3-4. Visualize fresh, clean energy flowing in through the top of your head and down through your body.
5 Breathe out 1-2-3-4. Visualize that clean energy driving all the dark feelings down and away through the soles of your feet.
6 Open your eyes.

Practising relaxation regularly will not only relieve stress but also increase your energy and focus and improve your problem-solving abilities.

6 Meditation

Calming the mind

Meditation has been around in many forms, religious and non-religious, for thousands of years. Its essence is calming the mind, either through **concentration** on a specific idea or by **blanking out** conscious, verbal thoughts. It takes time and practice to become an adept in any form of meditation, but you can quickly learn some **simple meditation techniques** that can help to lower stress.

> **'Calm the winds of your thoughts, and there will be no waves on the ocean of your mind.'**
>
> Anon.

Approaches to meditation

There are many approaches to meditation. For example, your **body** may be:

* sitting in a carefully defined posture
* sitting however you feel comfortable
* walking
* performing ritualized movements, e.g. yoga or tai chi.

Your **thoughts** may be:

* focused on a word of power
* focused on some aspect of your body
* open to the world around you.

Don't just do something – sit there!

The meditation posture

Adopting the **right posture** helps to focus the mind. You need to be upright – so you stay awake, and in balance. Sitting on a firm chair will do, but this is better:

1 Sit, on a cushion or a soft mat, upright with shoulders even and relaxed.
2 Cross your legs; the lotus position, with both feet up on the opposite thighs, is optional.
3 Hold your head up, with the chin tucked in a little to tilt the eyes down.
4 Have the eyes half shut, and unfocused.
5 Hold the mouth gently closed, with the tongue touching the upper teeth. This helps to reduce thirst.
6 Your hands can rest in your lap or on your knees, palms up or down. Do whatever is most comfortable.

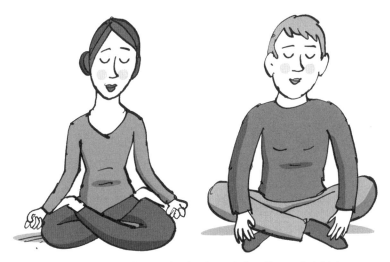

● The classic lotus posture (left) and a simpler variation. Be comfortable!

Mindful breathing

In Buddhism, **mindfulness** – being aware of yourself and your surroundings – is an essential step on the path to enlightenment. In the last few decades, this ancient concept and its practice have become accepted by Western medicine in the treatment of stress and anxiety, addictive behaviours such as obsessive-compulsive disorder and depression.

Like other forms of meditation, **mindful breathing** relieves stress by shutting out verbal thoughts. It allows you to focus your mind on the sensations of your body as it breathes.

> **'The breath is the connecting link between the inner world of the mind and the outer world of the body and environment.'**
>
> Sri Sri Ravi Shankar

66

Mindful breathing exercise

Allow 10 to 15 minutes for this.

1 Find a quiet place.
2 Sit in the meditation posture.
3 Breathe normally, but be aware of your breathing.
4 Feel the sensation of air in your nose, and the movements of your body.
5 If other thoughts come into your mind – and they will – do not fight them. Just acknowledge them, and then turn your focus back to your breathing.

Don't worry if you seem to be making slow progress in shutting out verbal thoughts. This is a practice, so don't expect it to be perfect straight away; the benefit is in the **practice**.

This is a practice, so don't expect it to be perfect straight away

Mindful walking

Mindfulness can be applied to walking and other activities. Mindful walking, also known as **walking meditation**, combines the benefits of exercise and meditation.

The aim is to be aware of the sensations of your body as it moves, and to **open up your senses** to the world around you. You shouldn't try to verbalize the sensations – just feel them.

Mindful walking is best done in the countryside, a park or a quiet street.

Top tip
Don't fight the ideas that pop into your head. Just don't dwell on them, but **refocus** on your breathing or walking. With practice, the awareness will push out the verbal thoughts.

Walking mindfully

* Make a **conscious decision** to start walking mindfully.
* Notice the **sensations** as you move your legs. Feel the muscles in action and the texture of the ground beneath your feet.
* Notice your **breathing**; feel and smell the air you breathe.
* Feel **the air on your skin** as you move.
* Open your senses to your **surroundings**, starting with those you normally use least.
* What can you smell? What can you hear? What can you see? **Take note**, but don't describe things to yourself. This is about avoiding verbal thoughts.
* When other thoughts and emotions intrude, acknowledge them, and then **bring your mind gently back to the walk**.

Mindful walking combines the benefits of exercise and meditation

Qi – the energy of life

Qi, the **life force**, is a central idea of Chinese medicine. In a healthy body it flows freely along its proper channels. **Acupuncture** aims to cure illness by regulating this flow. Qi (pronounced 'chee') can also be controlled through exercise and/or meditation in many ways, including:

* **Qi gong**
  » This is a form of breathing meditation where the arms and upper body move in rhythm with the breath.
* **Tai chi**
  » Movements based on martial arts are performed very slowly, with emphasis on balance, harmony and control.

In Maoist China 24-form tai chi was developed as exercises for the masses to encourage good health, and is now practised throughout the world.

70

Recharging the batteries

This quickly **restores calm** and **replenishes energy**. It helps if you visualize the qi while doing this – think of it as light.

1 Stand relaxed, legs slightly apart, head upright.
2 Begin with your arms by your sides, palms outwards.
3 Breathe in slowly, and as you do so sweep your arms up and over until the fingertips almost touch above your head. Visualize your hands gathering the qi.
4 Breathe out slowly, bringing your hands down, palms level, in front of you. Lower them down to your sides and turn the palms outwards. Visualize the qi entering through the top of your head and flooding through your body.
5 Repeat four or five times.

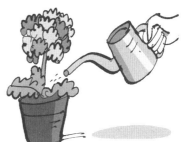

● Flood your body with energy

7 Why worry?

Worry and stress

Worry and stress may create **another vicious circle**. Stressful situations make us worry, but worrying adds to our stress by the tension it creates, and by interfering with our sleeping, eating and drinking habits.

The aim of this chapter is to help you **reduce your worrying** in the following stages:

* **Eliminate** most of your past and future worries.
* **Ignore** things that are not worth worrying about.
* **Think and act**, instead of worrying.

Worry can become a kind of **bad habit**, stopping us from getting on with what we really need to do.

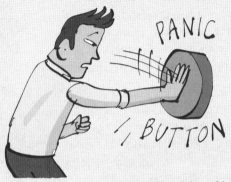

● 'I don't waste time worrying. When anything shows the slightest hint of going wrong, I jump straight into panic mode.'

Worry and stress are another vicious circle

Past, present and future worries

Whether the worry is about a relationship, work, money, your health or someone else's, the state of the world, or anything else, the focus of the worry is typically what you or another person **did, do or will do**, and the **impact** of that action.

We worry about things that have happened, are happening now, or that might happen. Past, present and future events need to be treated in different ways, but you can apply the **same approach** to every sort of worry.

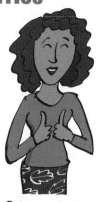

● 'No worries!'

'I'm an old man and I've had many troubles, most of which never happened.'

Mark Twain

Past

If it's completely over and done with – whether it's a broken teapot, cock-up at work, finished relationship – then:

1 Go over it carefully one last (really!) time and see what **lessons** can be learned in case a similar situation occurs in future.
2 **Put it away** and stop worrying about it.

If there are **consequences** to deal with, treat them as a present worry.

Future

1 If the event is highly unlikely and/or not likely to happen for a long time, **don't waste time** worrying about it.
2 Otherwise, treat it as a **present worry**, as action taken now can change the future.

Present

Put it through the **worry filter** – read on!

The worry filter

For this you need three jars and a handful of strips of paper, or a sheet of paper divided into three columns. Label the jars, or head up the columns, with:

Think (these are things you need to think more about)	Act (things you need to do something about)	Forget (stop worrying about it!)

Take each of your worries in turn, **process them** through the worry filter, then write them on a piece of paper and drop into the appropriate jar (or column).

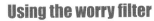

● Worry flow chart

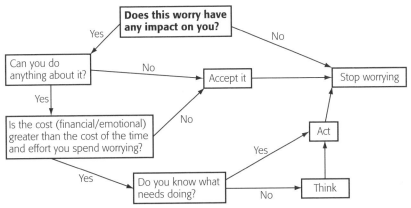

Does this worry have any impact on you?

Yes

No

Can you do anything about it?

No → Accept it

Stop worrying

Yes

Is the cost (financial/emotional) greater than the cost of the time and effort you spend worrying?

No

Act

Yes

Do you know what needs doing?

Yes

No → Think

79

Keep things in perspective!

Ask anyone who has **real problems**, or who has suffered real loss, and they will tell you that many things are not that important.

Think...

When you think something through, your thoughts move in one direction. They may branch off, loop or meander about, but eventually **reach their conclusion**. When you worry, your thoughts keep going over the same ground. To break out of the worry circle:

* **recognize** that you are in it, and not getting anywhere
* **focus** on the probable, the practical and the realistic
* **accept** that some things cannot be known in advance, and learn to live with uncertainty.

Don't worry through the night
Instead, write down your worries **before** you go to bed, and return to them in the morning when you are refreshed and better able to think things through.

...and act

There's nothing like **doing something** about it to solve a problem. You don't even need to solve it entirely. If you can reduce a problem, even by a very little, you'll feel more in control, and you will worry less.

* In a **difficult relationship**, can you talk to the other person about the issues?
* At **work**, can you improve your time management or work practices to reduce stresses?
* If the **size of a task** – at home or at work – is daunting, can you break it down into smaller parts?
* If **money** is a worry, is there any way to reduce outgoings or increase your income?

'Don't worry about a thing, 'cause every little thing's gonna be all right.'
Bob Marley

Accept the inevitable

If something is **totally beyond your control**, there's no point in worrying about it, no matter how big it is. At some point in the future, a giant asteroid is probably going to hit the Earth, but there's nothing you can do to stop it, so why worry?

More likely, a serious illness, redundancy or other unavoidable disaster may hit you or your family. As long as it's only a **possibility**, why worry? If it happens, there's even less point in worrying. Put your energies into the **good things** of your life and hang on to those. It's not easy – you may need help to get through.

As long as it's only a possibility, why worry?

Accepting uncertainty

You won't know what the new job, house, workmate or project will be like **until it happens.** You can't know how a difficult conversation will turn out until it starts. All very worrying? Not necessarily.

* If there's anything that you should be doing **in preparation**, do it.
* **Be open** in your expectations. If the future has to fit a certain mould, you are more likely to be disappointed, and to worry in advance.
* **Be hopeful.**

'If you can't fight or flee, let it flow.'

Anon.

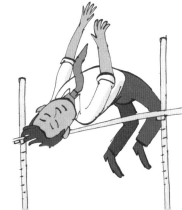

● 'I thought I'd just go with the flow.'

8 What really matters

Priorities and targets

It can take a little time and effort to sort out your **priorities** and **targets** for your daily life, and even more so for the longer term, but it's worth doing.

Clear targets reduce uncertainty and conflict – both sources of stress.

If you're working to your **priorities** and run short of time, it's the less important stuff that doesn't get done – and that's easier to live with.

Rule number 1: Your priorities must have top priority

In this chapter, we'll also talk about that elusive thing – the work–life balance. Getting that right at least most of the time can be the secret to a less stressful existence.

'In the long run, men only hit what they aim at.'
Henry David Thoreau

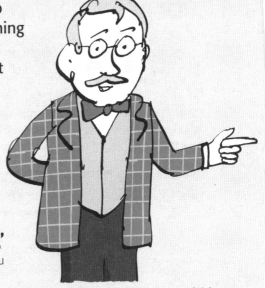

● 'Five years from now, I aim to be young, handsome and rich… On second thoughts, let's just start with my money-making plans.'

Your targets...

Take a little time out of your busy life to think about the following questions. And think about them on **two timescales** – the 10/20/30-year long term and the 1–5-year short term.

* What do you want out of your life?
* Is that different from what you have now?
* How can you best achieve the changes or maintain what you have?
* Which aspects of your future life are most important to you?

Always remember that you do not have to be driven. You do not have to achieve great heights. Being **happy** and **comfortable** is a valid life aim.

Top tip
Writing down your targets and priorities will help you clarify them.

...and priorities

Your targets are the things you aim to do or be; your priorities set the **order** in which you do things, and the amount of effort you put into them. They should arise from your targets. Take each of your targets in turn and ask these questions:

* What do I need to do to achieve this?
* What do I need to do first, then next?
* Will what I am doing now help me achieve this target?

> **'You've got to think about "big things" while you're doing small things, so that all the small things go in the right direction.'**
>
> Alvin Toffler

The work–life balance

There is no ideal, quantifiable, work–life balance – 50:50 or 80:20, or whatever. We each need to find **our own balance**, based partly on our targets and partly on the other people in our life, because they are part of the balance. You will find it useful to ask for their opinions when answering these questions with 'never', 'sometimes' or 'regularly'.

> *How often does your work interfere with your social/family/love life?*

> *How often does your outside life interfere with your job?*

In both cases, 'interfere with' may mean 'prevent you from being there when you are supposed to be' or 'occupy your thoughts so that you cannot participate properly'.

Finding the balance

If other people's answer to either question is 'regularly' – even though you would say 'sometimes' – you need to find **a better balance**, because the current one is causing you stress.

1 Think again about your targets. Are they **mutually compatible**? Which one is most important?
2 Compare your priorities for each target, looking for **clashes.** Are your career priorities clashing with those of your social or love life? Even if there is no actual clash, which priority should take precedence?
3 Try to identify **two or three achievable changes** to your routines that would help improve the balance.

We each need to find our own work–life balance

Whose priorities?

How far are your priorities **your own**? We all play **multiple roles** as workers, parents, partners, children, friends and members of other groups. All of these impose some priorities on us, and we must accept at least some of these to fulfil the roles properly.

If you feel that **other people's priorities** are pushing into the queue ahead of yours, it can be a source of stress. This may be most obvious at work.

Tasks should be prioritized in this order:

1 the **requirements** of your defined job
2 the **demands** of those higher up the line
3 the **requests** of colleagues.

But within that are different levels of priority.

Combining priorities

Don't let other people's high priorities push yours aside. Keep the job manageable by dealing with your own priorities first.

See 'How to say no at work' and 'How to say no to the boss' in chapter 10.

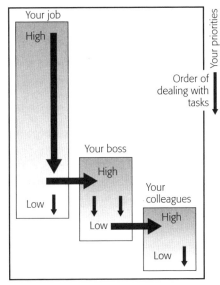

● Whose priority?

Urgent and important

There's a **big difference** between urgent and important.

* Urgent means it has to be done quickly.
* Important means it has to be done well.

When **setting priorities,** remember:

* Some urgent things are not important.
* Some important things are not urgent.

What is important and/or urgent to someone else may be neither to you.

> ### Top tip
> The way to get things done is to mitigate the urgent to spend more time on the important. This will help you achieve your goals better than dealing with a stream of urgent tasks.

When the jobs are piling up, assess the urgency and importance of each, then tackle them in the order listed in the table below. Make sure you allocate time for important jobs **when they first arrive**, even if you do not do them until later.

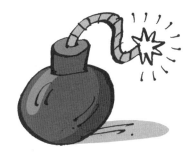

● If it's urgent and important, do it now!

Urgent and important	Important, not urgent	Urgent, not important	Not important, not urgent
1 Do this now!	2 Schedule time for this, then 4 Do it	3 Do this next	5 Does this need doing at all?

9 Time management

How long will it take?

Some jobs are of **known duration**: a three-hour training session, a one-day visit to a distant client. Others are **task-based**: researching and writing a report, decorating a birthday cake, carving a replacement table leg. Before you commit to the job, you need to assess how long it will take and check that you can fit it into your schedule.

This chapter offers practical techniques to help you do just that.

Always allow yourself enough time!

The five-minute (DIY) job

Anyone who has done any kind of DIY – mending a fuse, hanging a picture, fixing a dripping tap, or whatever – will recognize this.

A five-minute DIY job can only be done in five minutes if:

* you have all the tools and materials to hand at the start
* you really do know what you are doing
* nothing goes wrong
* nothing interrupts you
* the gods smile on you.

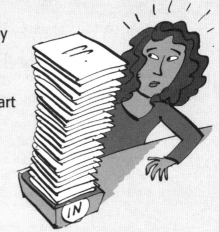

● This won't take five minutes!

Assessing the job

The need to allocate enough time to jobs is as true for little jobs as for big ones. Even a small job that overruns puts **your schedule under pressure,** and you under stress.

This is just as true for household tasks and family chores as for work projects.

Value your time – and yourself – properly

How much time do you need to do the job?

1 Have you done this before?
2 If so, allocate time by value.
3 How long did it take last time?
4 What's different this time? It should take as long as last time.
5 If there's more to do, allocate time by value to the extra work.

Adding extra time

When you've got a realistic estimate of the time, add on **extra time** for things going wrong. As a rough guide, add 10 per cent for simple jobs, and a further 10 per cent for every extra complexity or other person involved.

If the **worst** happens, you should still finish within the available time; if things go **smoothly** you will have spare time to put your feet up, or get on with something else.

Here's what your plan should look like:

Estimated time to do the job	Extra time
If all goes well…	Time limit

'Make use of time, let not advantage slip.'

William Shakespeare

Allocating time by value

You **have to do** some things just because you have to do them, but generally, you should allocate a value to a task – money saved or money earned. From that figure you can **calculate** how much time to allow for it.

1 Write down the value of the task.
2 Subtract the cost of materials needed for the job.
3 Divide by your hourly (or daily) rate. The result is the number of hours (or days) that can be spent on it.
4 If you have the time, and are confident it will be enough, take the job on.
5 If the time is not available or not long enough, don't do it.

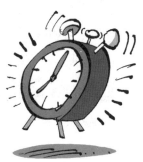

● If the time is not available, don't do it.

Nosnikrap's Wal

Parkinson's Law states:
'Work expands so as to fill the time available for its completion.'

Nosnikrap's Wal states:
'Work contracts to fit into the available time.'

And this is often true, especially with open-ended jobs. If you are asked to write a summary report on something that you know quite well – so you don't have to research it first – you could probably do just as good a job in two hours as in a whole day.

Doing things by halves

You have a deadline. Here's a **simple technique** to help ensure that the job is done in time.

1 Before you start, decide on the halfway marker for the job.
2 When you are halfway through the available time, check the job.
3 If you are less than halfway through it, take a few moments to reassess the job.
4 What can be simplified? What can be omitted? Can anyone else do part of it?
5 Set a new schedule, allowing the time to extend into some – not all – of the extra time.
6 Set a new marker for where you should be halfway through the remaining time
7 Repeat steps 2 and 3.

104

With more complex jobs and longer deadlines, set progress targets **at regular intervals** from early on to keep the job on track.

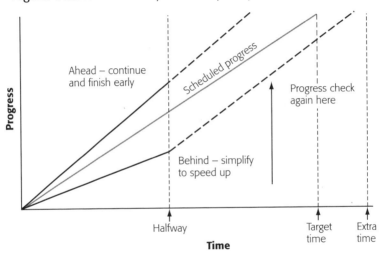

- Time–progress graph

Work smarter, not harder

Before you start any job, ask yourself this question:

Does this **really** need doing?

If the answer's yes, then ask yourself:

Am I the **best person** to do it?

Does it need more/fewer skills? Is there anyone else? If the answer's still yes, spend time preparing before you do anything.

* Look back at similar jobs you've done in the past. What can you learn from those?
* Think the job through in outline and decide the best way to tackle it.
* Now think through the details and see what you've missed.
* Work out the resources needed, and make sure they are available.
* Decide how you'll tell when the job is done.

When is the job done?

If you work for someone else, and a job is finished when the boss says it is, stop reading now.

With some jobs, the answer is simple: the car is repaired when it's working again; the database is up to date when all current data has been entered into it. Others may be harder to sign off. At what point do you stop rewriting a report? When are all the items in the display presented exactly right?

Nothing is ever perfect. If the job is done well enough to meet or exceed the boss's/client's/public's expectations, that's good enough.

> 'Give me six hours to chop down a tree, and I will spend the first four hours sharpening the axe.'
>
> Abraham Lincoln

10 The art of saying no

Knowing your limits

Saying no can be a great **stress reducer**. It frees up time that would be spent doing things that matter to other people, and leaves more time to do the things that matter to you.

If you are the sort of obliging person who likes to get on with other people, the prospect of saying no can be stressful – and we don't want that. Saying no does not have to be stressful, and gets **easier with practice**.

We all have limits to what we can do well without undue stress, and others may need to be told

Do you need to learn how to say no?

It's nice to be popular, and it's flattering when people see you as the one who can get things done, but sometimes it can get to be **too much**. You need to learn how to say no if:

* at work, you are struggling to find time to **complete** your own jobs
* at work or at home, you feel that you are doing more than your **fair share**
* in your social life, you agree to do things **you don't really want to do**.

This chapter tells you how to say no in these situations – and when to say yes.

How to say no at work

The next time someone asks you to do an extra chore for which you do not have time, say no. Follow these **guidelines**, and you can say no without getting stressed and without creating a stressful situation:

* **Refuse the request**, not the person. You are willing to help, but do not have the time.
* Refuse **with a smile**. There's no point in making enemies, and you may want their help another day.
* Make it clear that you have **your own priorities**. Your own work must come first.
* Make **helpful suggestions**, if you can.

Make helpful suggestions, if you can
. . . .

Examples:

* 'Sorry, I'd love to help, but I really don't have time right now...'
* 'Sorry, but I must get this finished before I can do anything else...'
* 'Have you asked Bob? He may be able to help...'
* 'It's simple if you use XYZ software. Get Tech Support to show you how...'

If they persist in the request, persist in the refusal and **stick to your guns**:

* 'No, really, I do not have the time...'
* 'This job must take priority...'
* 'It may only be a ten-minute job, but I don't have even five minutes to spare...'

Keep calm
If you feel yourself getting angry at someone's inability to take 'no' for an answer, stop, count down from ten, calm down, and refuse again – with a smile.

How to say no to the boss

This can be tricky, because:

* you shouldn't be refusing any **reasonable request**
* you may not want to admit that you **can't cope** with the job.

But if you don't say 'Stop!' now and then, your boss may keep piling on the work simply because he or she thinks you are coping happily.

Before it gets too much, ask for a **meeting**. Keep calm, be reasonable, be helpful, but **be realistic** about the limitations of time and energy. The boss may have unrealistic ideas about how long things take to do. You may be overworking – giving jobs a higher level of detail and finish than they need.

You need to clarify expectations

What is expected of you?

You need to clarify other people's expectations.

* **How much work** are you expected to do?
* **How much time** are jobs expected to take?
* If the task is over and above your normal workload, what other work is to be omitted or delayed to make way for it?

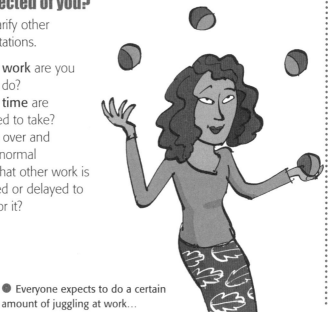

115

● Everyone expects to do a certain amount of juggling at work…

How to say no to friends and family

Unwanted invitations

* First rule, start by **thanking** them for the offer.
* Give a **good reason** for refusing, but only one. If you give more than one reason, they'll be taken as excuses.
* If you want to, then leave open the possibility of saying yes **another time**:
    » 'Thank you, but I've already got plans for that day…'
    » 'Thank you, but I don't want to see that film…'
    » 'Thank you, but that would finish too late for me.'
* If they persist, **repeat the refusal,** perhaps using different words but with the same message:
    » 'Sorry no, I've already agreed to be elsewhere…'
    » 'No thanks, I read the review and I know I won't enjoy it…'
    » 'I have an early start tomorrow, so I need to get some rest.'

Excessive demands

Mutual help and co-operation are the essence of friendship and family life, but it's two-way. If you feel that you are being put upon or asked to do more than your fair share of chores, use the same techniques as for saying no at work. It is important to try to make your stand before resentment damages relationships.

'Half of the troubles of this life can be traced to saying yes too quickly and not saying no soon enough.'
Josh Billings

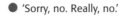

● 'Sorry, no. Really, no.'

When to say yes

You're scurrying around, struggling to get things done, time's running out, and someone says, 'Do you want a hand?' What's stopping you from saying yes?

I don't say yes because:

It will take longer to show them how to do it than to do it myself.

They won't do it as well as I will.

I don't want to owe them a favour.

I don't want people to think I need help.

Why that's a bad reason

It may be true this time, but next time they will know how.

They will if you give them a chance to practise.

They are your colleagues/ friends/family – you are supposed to co-operate.

Everyone knows how much you achieve by yourself. You don't need to prove it.

A common reason for stress is the urge to do everything yourself, but you will be the loser in the long run.

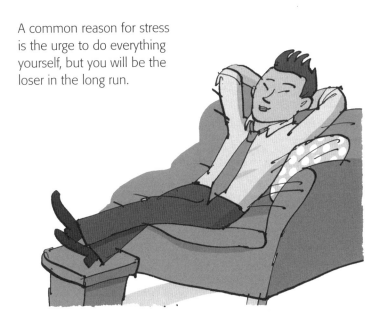

● 'How beautiful it is to do nothing, and then to rest afterward.' (Spanish proverb)

What next?

In this book I have tried to give some straightforward techniques to help you cope better with stress. I hope that your life is not too stressful, and that these techniques will be enough, but if not, you may find these books and websites useful:

Gunaratana, Henepola, *Mindfulness in Plain English* (Somerville: Wisdom Publications, 2002)

Looker, Terry, *Manage Your Stress for a Happier Life: Teach Yourself* (London: Hodder Education, 2011)

The Stress Management Society at stress.org.uk

The Royal College of Psychiatrists at rcpsych.ac.uk

The US National Library of medicine at nlm.nih.gov

The health information site familydoctor.org also has articles on coping with stress.